The Ultimate Air Fryer Breakfast Cooking Guide

Easy And Healthy Air Fryer Breakfast Recipes For Beginners

Ellie Sloan

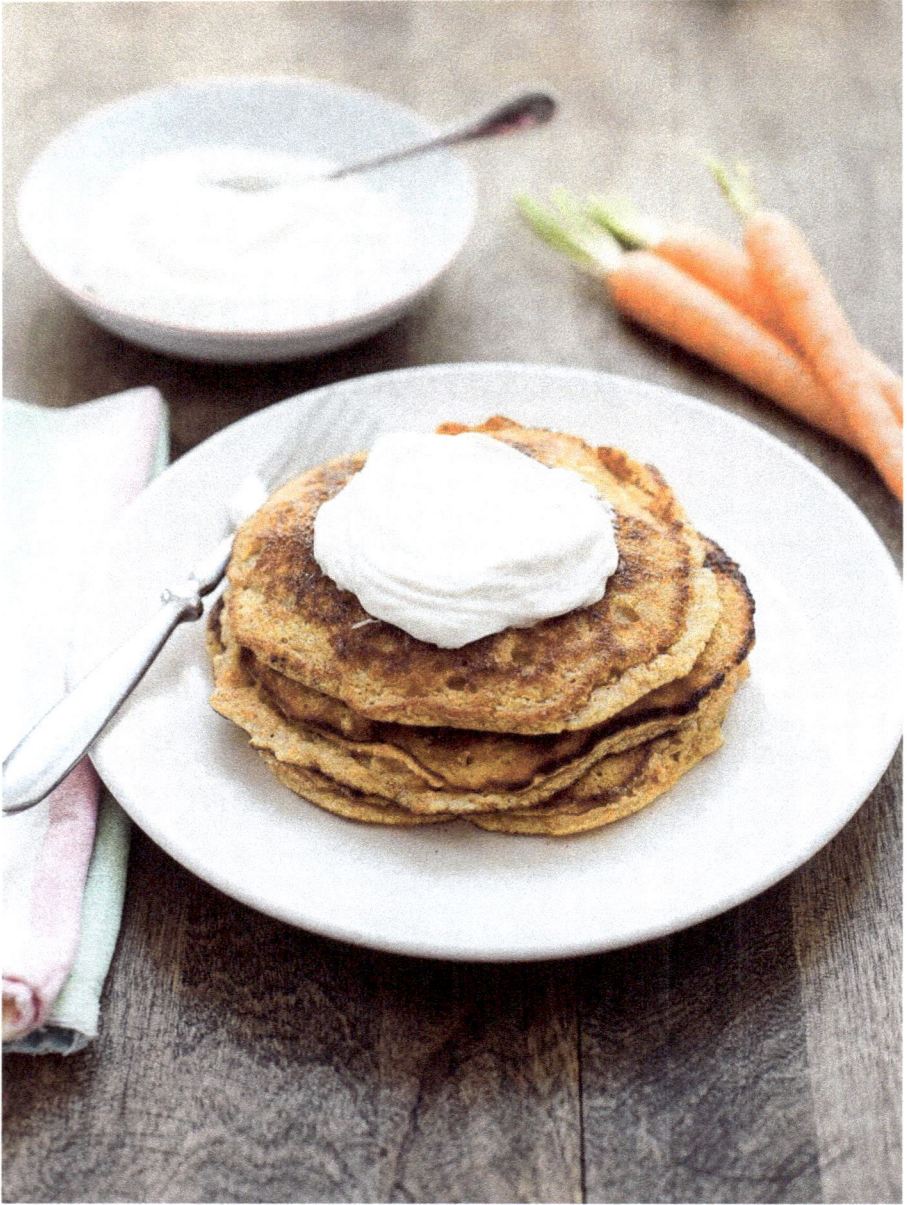

Table of contents

Zucchini Muffins

Preparation Time: 10 minutes

Cooking Time: 20 minutes

Servings: 8

Ingredients:

- 6 eggs
- 4 drops stevia
- 1/4 cup swerve
- 1/3 cup coconut oil, melted
- 1 cup zucchini, grated
- 3/4 cup coconut flour
- 1/4 tsp. ground nutmeg
- 1 tsp. ground cinnamon
- 1/2 tsp. baking soda

Directions:

1. Preheat the Air Fryer to 325°F.
2. Add all ingredients except zucchini in a bowl and mix well.
3. Add zucchini and stir well.

4. Pour batter into the silicone muffin molds and place into the Air Fryer basket.
5. Cook muffins for 20 minutes
6. Serve and enjoy.

Nutrition:

Calories 136, Fat 12g, Carbs 1g, Protein 4g

Jalapeno Breakfast Muffins

Preparation Time: 10 minutes

Cooking Time: 15 minutes

Servings: 8

Ingredients:

- 5 eggs
- 1/3 cup coconut oil, melted
- 2 tsp. baking powder
- 3 tbsp. erythritol
- 3 tbsp. jalapenos, sliced
- 1/4 cup unsweetened coconut milk
- 2/3 cup coconut flour
- 3/4 tsp. sea salt

Directions:

1. Preheat the Air Fryer to 325°F.
2. In a large bowl, mix together coconut flour, baking powder, erythritol, and sea salt.
3. Stir in eggs, jalapenos, coconut milk, and coconut oil until well combined.

4. Pour batter into the silicone muffin molds and place into the Air Fryer basket.
5. Cook muffins for 15 minutes
6. Serve and enjoy.

Nutrition:

Calories 125, Fat 12g, Carbs 7g, Protein 3g

Simple Egg Soufflé

Preparation Time: 5 minutes

Cooking Time: 8 minutes

Servings: 2

Ingredients:

- 2 eggs
- 1/4 tsp. chili pepper
- 2 tbsp. heavy cream
- 1/4 tsp. pepper
- 1 tbsp. parsley, chopped
- Salt

Directions:

1. In a bowl, whisk eggs with remaining gradients.
2. Spray two ramekins with cooking spray.
3. Pour egg mixture into the prepared ramekins and place into the Air Fryer basket.
4. Cook soufflé at 390°F for 8 minutes
5. Serve and enjoy.

Nutrition:

Calories 116, Fat 10g, Carbs 1.1g, Protein 6g

Vegetable Egg Soufflé

Preparation Time: 10 minutes

Cooking Time: 20 minutes

Servings: 4

Ingredients:

- 4 large eggs
- 1 tsp. onion powder
- 1 tsp. garlic powder
- 1 tsp. red pepper, crushed
- 1/2 cup broccoli florets, chopped
- 1/2 cup mushrooms, chopped

Directions:

1. Sprinkle four ramekins with cooking spray and set aside.
2. In a bowl, whisk eggs with onion powder, garlic powder, and red pepper.
3. Add mushrooms and broccoli and stir well.
4. Pour egg mixture into the prepared ramekins and place ramekins into the Air Fryer basket.

5. Cook at 350°F for 15 minutes. Make sure soufflé is cooked. If soufflé is not cooked, then cook for 5 minutes more.
6. Serve and enjoy.

Nutrition:

Calories 91, Fat 5.1g, Carbs 4.7g, Protein 7.4g

Asparagus Frittata

Preparation Time: 10 minutes

Cooking Time: 10 minutes

Servings: 4

Ingredients:

- 6 eggs
- 3 mushrooms, sliced
- 10 asparagus, chopped
- 1/4 cup half and half
- 2 tsp. butter, melted
- 1 cup mozzarella cheese, shredded
- 1 tsp. pepper
- 1 tsp. salt

Directions:

1. Toss mushrooms and asparagus with melted butter and add into the Air Fryer basket. Cook mushrooms and asparagus at 350°F for 5 minutes. Shake basket twice.

2. Meanwhile, in a bowl, whisk together eggs, half and half, pepper, and salt. Transfer cook mushrooms and asparagus into the Air Fryer baking dish. Pour egg mixture over mushrooms and asparagus.

3. Place dish in the Air Fryer and cook at 350°F for 5 minutes or until eggs are set. Slice and serve.

Nutrition:

Calories 211, Fat 13g, Carbs 4g, Protein 16g

Spicy Cauliflower Rice

Preparation Time: 10 minutes

Cooking Time: 22 minutes

Servings: 2

Ingredients:

- 1 cauliflower head, cut into florets
- 1/2 tsp. cumin
- 1/2 tsp. chili powder
- 6 onion spring, chopped
- 2 jalapenos, chopped
- 4 tbsp. olive oil
- 1 zucchini, trimmed and cut into cubes
- 1/2 tsp. paprika
- 1/2 tsp. garlic powder
- 1/2 tsp. cayenne pepper
- 1/2 tsp. pepper
- 1/2 tsp. salt

Directions:

1. Preheat the Air Fryer to 370°F.

2. Add cauliflower florets into the food processor and process until it looks like rice.

3. Transfer cauliflower rice into the Air Fryer baking pan and drizzle with half oil.

4. Place pan in the Air Fryer and cook for 12 minutes, stir halfway through.

5. Heat the remaining oil in a small pan over medium heat.

6. Add zucchini and cook for 5-8 minutes

7. Add onion and jalapenos and cook for 5 minutes

8. Add spices and stir well. Set aside.

9. Add cauliflower rice in the zucchini mixture and stir well.

10. Serve and enjoy.

Nutrition:

Calories 254, Fat 28g, Carbs 12.3g, Protein 4.3g

Broccoli Stuffed Peppers

Preparation Time: 10 minutes

Cooking Time: 40 minutes

Servings: 2

Ingredients:

- 4 eggs
- 1/2 cup cheddar cheese, grated
- 2 bell peppers cut in half and remove seeds
- 1/2 tsp. garlic powder
- 1 tsp. dried thyme
- 1/4 cup feta cheese, crumbled
- 1/2 cup broccoli, cooked
- 1/4 tsp. pepper
- 1/2 tsp. salt

Directions:

1. Preheat the Air Fryer to 325°F.
2. Stuff feta and broccoli into the bell peppers halved.
3. Beat egg in a bowl with seasoning and pour egg mixture into the pepper halved over feta and broccoli.

4. Place bell pepper halved into the Air Fryer basket and cook for 35-40 minutes
5. Top with grated cheddar cheese and cook until cheese melted.
6. Serve and enjoy.

Nutrition:

Calories 340, Fat 22g, Carbs 12g, Protein 22g

Zucchini Noodles

Preparation Time: 10 minutes

Cooking Time: 44 minutes

Servings: 3

Ingredients:

- 1 egg
- 1/2 cup parmesan cheese, grated
- 1/2 cup feta cheese, crumbled
- 1 tbsp. thyme
- 1 garlic clove, chopped
- 1 onion, chopped
- 2 medium zucchinis, trimmed and spiralized
- 2 tbsp. olive oil
- 1 cup mozzarella cheese, grated
- 1/2 tsp. pepper
- 1/2 tsp. salt

Directions:

1. Preheat the Air Fryer to 350°F.

2. Add spiralized zucchini and salt in a colander and set aside for 10 minutes. Wash zucchini noodles and pat dry with a paper towel.

3. Heat the oil in a pan over medium heat. Add garlic and onion and sauté for 3-4 minutes

4. Add zucchini noodles and cook for 4-5 minutes or until softened.

5. Add zucchini mixture into the Air Fryer baking pan. Add egg, thyme, cheeses. Mix well and season.

6. Place pan in the Air Fryer and cook for 30-35 minutes

7. Serve and enjoy.

Nutrition:

Calories 435, Fat 29g, Carbs 10.4g, Protein 25g

Mushroom Frittata

Preparation Time: 10 minutes

Cooking Time: 13 minutes

Servings: 1

Ingredients:

- 1 cup egg whites
- 1 cup spinach, chopped
- 2 mushrooms, sliced
- 2 tbsp. parmesan cheese, grated
- Salt

Directions:

1. Sprinkle pan with cooking spray and heat over medium heat. Add mushrooms and sauté for 2-3 minutes Add spinach and cook for 1-2 minutes or until wilted.
2. Transfer mushroom spinach mixture into the Air Fryer pan. Beat egg whites in a mixing bowl until frothy. Season it with a pinch of salt.

3. Pour egg white mixture into the spinach and mushroom mixture and sprinkle with parmesan cheese. Place pan in Air Fryer basket and cook frittata at 350°F for 8 minutes
4. Slice and serve.

Nutrition:

Calories 176, Fat 3g, Carbs 4g, Protein 31g

Blueberry Breakfast Cobbler

Preparation Time: 5 minutes

Cooking Time: 15 minutes

Servings: 4

Ingredients:

- ⅓ cup whole-wheat pastry flour
- ¾ tsp. baking powder
- Dash sea salt
- ½ cup 2% milk
- 2 tbsp. pure maple syrup
- ½ tsp. vanilla extract
- Cooking oil spray
- ½ cup fresh blueberries
- ¼ cup Granola, or plain store-bought granola

Directions:

1. In a medium bowl, whisk the flour, baking powder, and salt. Add the milk, maple syrup, and vanilla and gently whisk, just until thoroughly combined.

2. Preheat the unit in bake mode, setting the temperature to 350°F, and setting the time to 3 minutes.

3. Spray a 6-by-2-inch round baking pan with cooking oil and pour the batter into the pan. Top evenly with the blueberries and granola.

4. Once the unit is preheated, place the pan into the basket and cook for 15 minutes.

5. When the cooking is complete, the cobbler should be nicely browned and a knife inserted into the middle should come out clean. Enjoy plain or topped with a little vanilla yogurt.

Nutrition:

Calories 112, Fat 1g, Carbs 23g, Protein 3g

Yummy Breakfast Italian Frittata

Preparation Time: 5 minutes

Cooking Time: 10 minutes

Servings: 6

Ingredients:

- 6 eggs
- 1/3 cup of milk
- 4 oz. of chopped Italian sausage
- 3 cups of stemmed and roughly chopped kale
- 1 red deseeded and chopped bell pepper
- ½ cup of a grated feta cheese
- 1 chopped zucchini
- 1 tbsp. of freshly chopped basil
- 1 tsp. of garlic powder
- 1 tsp. of onion powder
- 1 tsp. of salt
- 1 tsp. of black pepper

Directions:

1. Turn on your Air Fryer to 360°F.

2. Grease the Air Fryer pan with a nonstick cooking spray.
3. Add the Italian sausage to the pan and cook it inside your Air Fryer for 5 minutes
4. While doing that, add and stir in the remaining ingredients until it mixes properly.
5. Add the egg mixture to the pan and allow it to cook inside your Air Fryer for 5 minutes
6. Thereafter carefully remove the pan and allow it to cool off until it gets chill enough to serve.
7. Serve and enjoy!

Nutrition:

Calories 225, Fat 14g, Carbs 4.5g, Protein 20g

Savory Cheese and Bacon Muffins

Preparation Time: 5 minutes

Cooking Time: 17 minutes

Servings: 4

Ingredients:

- 1 ½ cup of all-purpose flour
- 2 tsp.s of baking powder
- ½ cup of milk
- 2 eggs
- 1 tbsp. of freshly chopped parsley
- 4 cooked and chopped bacon slices
- 1 thinly chopped onion
- ½ cup of shredded cheddar cheese
- ½ tsp. of onion powder
- 1 tsp. of salt
- 1 tsp. of black pepper

Directions:

1. Turn on your Air Fryer to 360°F.

2. Using a large bowl, add and stir all the ingredients until it mixes properly.
3. Then grease the muffin cups with a nonstick cooking spray or line it with a parchment paper. Pour the batter proportionally into each muffin cup.
4. Place it inside your Air Fryer and bake it for 15 minutes
5. Thereafter, carefully remove it from your Air Fryer and allow it to chill.
6. Serve and enjoy!

Nutrition:

Calories 180, Fat 18g, Carbs 16g, Protein 15g

Best Air-Fried English Breakfast

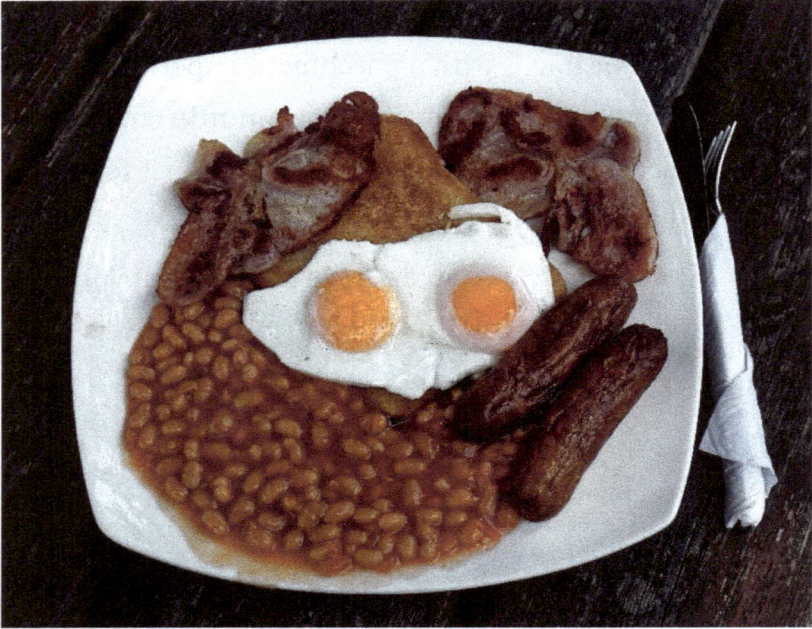

Preparation Time: 5 minutes

Cooking Time: 20 minutes

Servings: 4

Ingredients:

- 8 sausages
- 8 bacon slices
- 4 eggs

- 1 (16-oz.) can of baked beans
- 8 slices of toast

Directions:

1. Add the sausages and bacon slices to your Air Fryer and cook them for 10 minutes at a 320°F.
2. Using a ramekin or heat-safe bowl, add the baked beans, then place another ramekin and add the eggs and whisk.
3. Place it inside your Air Fryer and cook it for an additional 10 minutes or until everything is done.
4. Serve and enjoy!

Nutrition:

Calories 850, Fat 40g, Carbs 20g, Protein 48g

Sausage and Egg Breakfast Burrito

Preparation Time: 5 minutes

Cooking Time: 30 minutes

Servings: 6

Ingredients:

- 6 eggs
- Salt
- Pepper
- Cooking oil
- ½ cup chopped red bell pepper
- ½ cup chopped green bell pepper
- 8 oz. ground chicken sausage
- ½ cup salsa
- 6 medium (8-inch) flour tortillas
- ½ cup shredded Cheddar cheese

Directions:

1. In a medium bowl, whisk the eggs. Add salt and pepper to taste.

2. Place a skillet on medium-high heat. Spray with cooking oil. Add the eggs. Scramble for 2 to 3 minutes, until the eggs are fluffy. Remove the eggs from the skillet and set aside.

3. If needed, spray the skillet with more oil. Add the chopped red and green bell peppers. Cook for 2 to 3 minutes, once the peppers are soft.

4. Add the ground sausage to the skillet. Break the sausage into smaller pieces using a spatula or spoon. Cook for 3 to 4 minutes, until the sausage is brown.

5. Add the salsa and scrambled eggs. Stir to combine. Remove the skillet from heat.

6. Spoon the mixture evenly onto the tortillas.

7. To form the burritos, fold the sides of each tortilla in toward the middle and then roll up from the bottom. You can secure each burrito with a toothpick. Or you can moisten the outside edge of the tortilla with a small amount of water. I prefer to use a cooking brush, but you can also dab with your fingers.

8. Spray the burritos with cooking oil and place them in the Air Fryer. Do not stack. Cook the burritos in batches if they do not all fit in the basket. Cook for 8 minutes at 345°F

9. Open the Air Fryer and flip the burritos. Heat it for an additional 2 minutes or until crisp.

10. If necessary, repeat steps 8 and 9 for the remaining burritos.
11. Sprinkle the Cheddar cheese over the burritos. Cool before serving.

Nutrition:

Calories 236, Fat 13g, Carbs 16g, Protein 15g

French Toast Sticks

Preparation Time: 5 minutes

Cooking Time: 15 minutes

Servings: 12

Ingredients:

- 4 slices Texas toast (or any thick bread, such as challah)
- 1 tbsp. butter
- 1 egg
- 1 tsp. stevia
- 1 tsp. ground cinnamon
- ¼ cup milk
- 1 tsp. vanilla extract
- Cooking oil

Directions:

1. Cut each slice of bread into 3 pieces (for 12 sticks total).
2. Place the butter in a small, microwave-safe bowl. Heat for 15 seconds, or until the butter has melted.

3. Remove the bowl from the microwave. Add the egg, stevia, cinnamon, milk, and vanilla extract. Whisk until fully combined.
4. Sprinkle the Air Fryer basket with cooking oil.
5. Dredge each of the bread sticks in the egg mixture.
6. Place the French toast sticks in the Air Fryer. It is okay to stack them. Spray the French toast sticks with cooking oil. Cook for 8 minutes at 330°F
7. Open the Air Fryer and flip each of the French toast sticks. Cook for an additional 4 minutes, or until the French toast sticks are crisp.
8. Cool before serving.

Nutrition:

Calories 52, Fat 2g, Carbs 7g, Protein 2g

Home-Fried Potatoes

Preparation Time: 5 minutes

Cooking Time: 25 minutes

Servings: 4

Ingredients:

- 3 large russet potatoes
- 1 tbsp. canola oil
- 1 tbsp. extra-virgin olive oil
- 1 tsp. paprika
- Salt
- Pepper
- 1 cup chopped onion
- 1 cup chopped red bell pepper
- 1 cup chopped green bell pepper

Directions:

1. Cut the potatoes into ½-inch cubes. Place the potatoes in a large bowl of cold water and allow them to soak for at least 30 minutes, preferably an hour.

2. Dry out the potatoes and wipe thoroughly with paper towels. Return them to the empty bowl.

3. Add the canola and olive oils, paprika, and salt and pepper to flavor. Toss to fully coat the potatoes.

4. Transfer the potatoes to the Air Fryer. Cook for 20 minutes at 350°F, shaking the Air Fryer basket every 5 minutes (a total of 4 times).

5. Put the onion and red and green bell peppers to the Air Fryer basket. Fry for an additional 3 to 4 minutes, or until the potatoes are cooked through and the peppers are soft.

6. Cool before serving.

Nutrition:

Calories 279, Fat 8g, Carbs 50g, Protein 6g

Homemade Cherry Breakfast Tarts

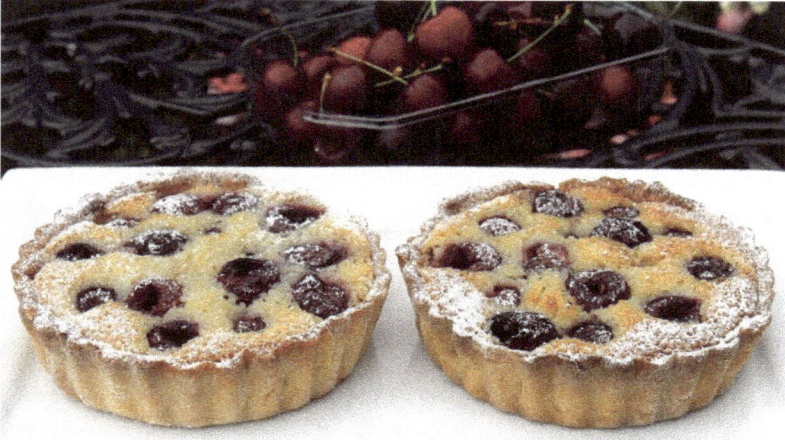

Preparation Time: 15 minutes

Cooking Time: 20 minutes

Servings: 6

Ingredients:

For the tarts:

- 2 refrigerated piecrusts
- ⅓ Cup cherry preserves
- 1 tsp. cornstarch
- Cooking oil

For the frosting:

- ½ cup vanilla yogurt
- 1 oz. cream cheese
- 1 tsp. stevia
- Rainbow sprinkles

Directions:

To make the tarts:

1. Place the piecrusts on a flat surface. Make use of a knife or pizza cutter, cut each piecrust into 3 rectangles, for 6 in total. (I discard the unused dough left from slicing the edges.)
2. In a small bowl, combine the preserves and cornstarch. Mix well.
3. Scoop 1 tbsp. of the preserve mixture onto the top half of each piece of piecrust.
4. Fold the bottom of each piece up to close the tart. Press along the edges of each tart to seal using the back of a fork.
5. Sprinkle the breakfast tarts with cooking oil and place them in the Air Fryer. I do not recommend piling the breakfast tarts. They will stick together if piled. You may need to prepare them in two batches. Cook for 10 minutes at 350°F

6. Allow the breakfast tarts to cool fully before removing from the Air Fryer.

7. If needed, repeat steps 5 and 6 for the remaining breakfast tarts.

To make the frosting:

8. In a small bowl, mix the yogurt, cream cheese, and stevia. Mix well.

9. Spread the breakfast tarts with frosting and top with sprinkles, and serve.

Nutrition:

Calories 119, Fat 4g, Carbs 19g, Protein 2g

Sausage and Cream Cheese Biscuits

Preparation Time: 5 minutes

Cooking Time: 15 minutes

Serving: 5

Ingredients:

- 12 oz. chicken breakfast sausage
- 1 (6 oz.) can biscuits
- ⅛ cup cream cheese

Directions:

1. Form the sausage into 5 small patties.
2. Place the sausage patties in the Air Fryer. Cook for 5 minutes a at 360°F
3. Open the Air Fryer. Flip the patties. Cook for an additional 5 minutes
4. Remove the cooked sausages from the Air Fryer.
5. Separate the biscuit dough into 5 biscuits.
6. Place the biscuits in the Air Fryer. Cook for 3 minutes
7. Open the Air Fryer. Flip the biscuits. Cook for an additional 2 minutes

8. Remove the cooked biscuits from the Air Fryer.

9. Split each biscuit in half. Spread 1 tsp. of cream cheese onto the bottom of each biscuit. Top with a sausage patty and the other half of the biscuit, and serve.

Nutrition:

Calories 240, Fat 13g, Carbs 20g, Protein 9g

Fried Chicken and Waffles

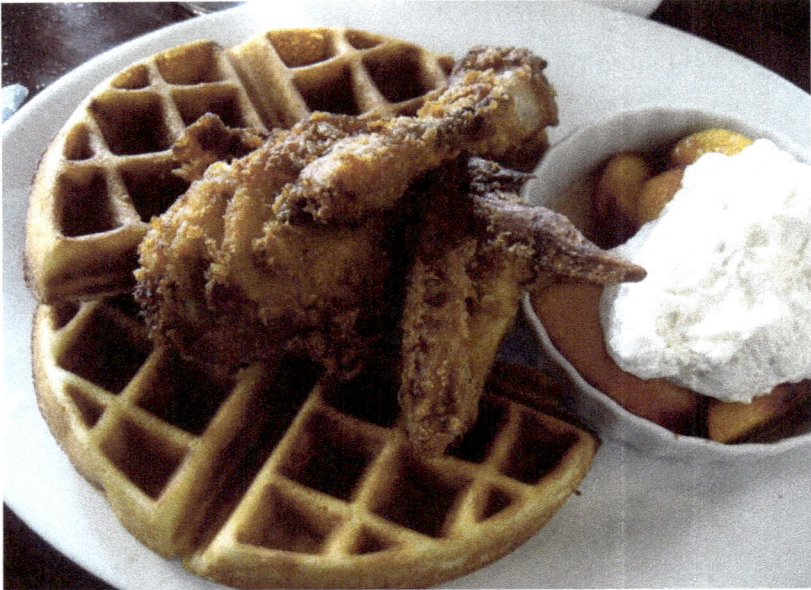

Preparation Time: 10 minutes

Cooking Time: 30 minutes

Servings: 4

Ingredients:

- 8 whole chicken wings
- 1 tsp. garlic powder
- Chicken seasoning or rub

- Pepper
- ½ cup all-purpose flour
- Cooking oil
- 8 frozen waffles
- Maple syrup (optional)

Directions:

1. In a medium bowl, spice the chicken with the garlic powder and chicken seasoning and pepper to flavor.
2. Put the chicken to a sealable plastic bag and add the flour. Shake to thoroughly coat the chicken.
3. Sprinkle the Air Fryer basket with cooking oil.
4. With the use of tongs, put the chicken from the bag to the Air Fryer. It is okay to pile the chicken wings on top of each other. Sprinkle them with cooking oil. Heat for five minutes at 380°F
5. Unlock the Air Fryer and shake the basket. Presume to cook the chicken. Keep shaking every 5 minutes until 20 minutes has passed and the chicken is completely cooked.
6. Take out the cooked chicken from the Air Fryer and set aside.
7. Wash the basket and base out with warm water. Put them back to the Air Fryer.

8. Ease the temperature of the Air Fryer to 370°F.
9. Put the frozen waffles in the Air Fryer. Do not pile. Depends on how big your Air Fryer is, you may need to cook the waffles in batches. Sprinkle the waffles with cooking oil. Cook for 6 minutes
10. If necessary, take out the cooked waffles from the Air Fryer, then repeat step 9 for the leftover waffles.
11. Serve the waffles with the chicken and a bit of maple syrup if desired.

Nutrition:

Calories 461, Fat 22g, Carbs 45g, Protein 28g

Cheesy Tater Tot Breakfast Bake

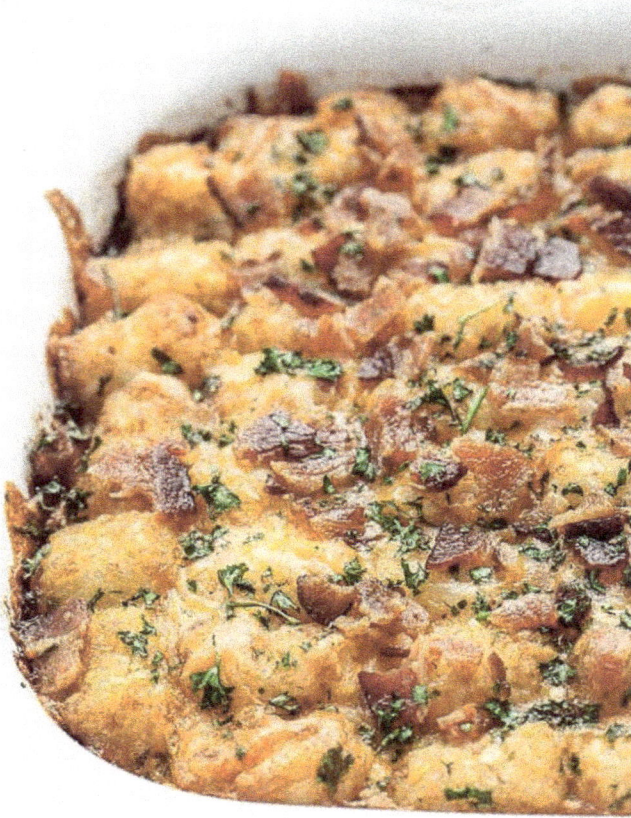

Preparation Time: 5 minutes

Cooking Time: 20 minutes

Servings: 4

Ingredients:

- 4 eggs
- 1 cup milk
- 1 tsp. onion powder
- Salt
- Pepper
- Cooking oil
- 12 oz. ground chicken sausage
- 1-lb. frozen tater tots
- ¾ cup shredded Cheddar cheese

Directions:

1. In a medium bowl, whisk the eggs. Add the milk, onion powder, and salt and pepper to taste. Stir to combine.
2. Spray a skillet with cooking oil and set over medium-high heat. Add the ground sausage. Using a spatula or spoon, break the sausage into smaller pieces. Cook for 3 to 4 minutes at 360°F, until the sausage is brown. Remove from heat and set aside.
3. Spray a barrel pan with cooking oil. Make sure to cover the bottom and sides of the pan. Place the tater tots in the barrel pan. Cook for 6 minutes

4. Open the Air Fryer and shake the pan, then add the egg mixture and cooked sausage. Cook for an additional 6 minutes. Open the Air Fryer and sprinkle the cheese over the tater tot bake. Cook for an additional 2 to 3 minutes. Cool before serving.

Nutrition:

Calories 518, Fat 30g, Carbs 31g, Protein 30g

Breakfast Scramble Casserole

Preparation Time: 20 minutes

Cooking Time: 10 minutes

Servings: 4

Ingredients:

- 6 slices bacon
- 6 eggs
- Salt
- Pepper
- Cooking oil
- ½ cup chopped red bell pepper
- ½ cup chopped green bell pepper
- ½ cup chopped onion
- ¾ cup shredded Cheddar cheese

Directions:

1. In a pan, over medium-high heat, cook the bacon, 5 to 7 minutes, flipping to evenly crisp. Dry out on paper towels, crumble, and set aside. In a medium bowl, whisk the eggs. Add salt and pepper to taste.

2. Spray a barrel pan with cooking oil. Make sure to cover the bottom and sides of the pan. Add the beaten eggs, crumbled bacon, red bell pepper, green bell pepper, and onion to the pan. Place the pan in the Air Fryer and cook for 6 minutes at 380°F. Open the Air Fryer and sprinkle the cheese over the casserole. Cook for an additional 2 minutes. Cool before serving.

Nutrition:

Calories 348, Fat 26g, Carbs 4g, Protein 25g

Breakfast Grilled Ham and Cheese

Preparation Time: 5 minutes

Cooking Time: 10 minutes

Servings: 2

Ingredients:

- 1 tsp. butter
- 4 slices bread
- 4 slices smoked country ham
- 4 slices Cheddar cheese
- 4 thick slices tomato

Directions:

1. Spread ½ tsp. of butter onto one side of 2 slices of bread. Each sandwich will have 1 slice of bread with butter and 1 slice without.
2. Assemble each sandwich by layering 2 slices of ham, 2 slices of cheese, and 2 slices of tomato on the unbuttered pieces of bread. Top with the other bread slices, buttered side up.

3. Place the sandwiches in the Air Fryer buttered-side down. Cook for 4 minutes at 330°F

4. Open the Air Fryer. Flip the grilled cheese sandwiches. Cook for an additional 4 minutes

5. Cool before serving. Cut each sandwich in half and enjoy.

Nutrition:

Calories 525,Fat 25g,Carbs 34g,Protein 41g

Classic Hash Browns

Preparation Time: 15 minutes

Cooking Time: 20 minutes

Servings: 4

Ingredients:

- 4 russet potatoes
- 1 tsp. paprika
- Salt
- Pepper
- Cooking oil

Directions:

1. Peel the potatoes using a vegetable peeler. Using a cheese grater shred the potatoes. If your grater has different-size holes, use the area of the tool with the largest holes.
2. Put the shredded potatoes in a large bowl of cold water. Let sit for 5 minutes Cold water helps remove excess starch from the potatoes. Stir to help dissolve the starch.

3. Dry out the potatoes and dry with paper towels or napkins. Make sure the potatoes are completely dry.
4. Season the potatoes with the paprika and salt and pepper to taste.
5. Spray the potatoes with cooking oil and transfer them to the Air Fryer. Cook for 20 minutes at 360°F and shake the basket every 5 minutes (a total of 4 times).
6. Cool before serving.

Nutrition:

Calories 150, Fat 9g, Carbs 34g, Protein 4g

Canadian Bacon and Cheese English Muffins

Preparation Time: 5 minutes

Cooking Time: 10 minutes

Servings: 4

Ingredients:

- 4 English muffins
- 8 slices Canadian bacon
- 4 slices cheese
- Cooking oil

Directions:

1. Split each English muffin. Assemble the breakfast sandwiches by layering 2 slices of Canadian bacon and 1 slice of cheese onto each English muffin bottom. Put the other half on top of the English muffin. Place the sandwiches in the Air Fryer. Spray the top of each with cooking oil. Cook for 4 minutes at 380°F

2. Open the Air Fryer and flip the sandwiches. Cook for an additional 4 minutes
3. Cool before serving.

Nutrition:

Calories 333, Fat 14g, Carbs 27g, Protein 24g

Radish Hash Browns

Preparation Time: 10 minutes

Cooking Time: 13 minutes

Servings: 4

Ingredients:

- 1 lb. radishes, washed and cut off roots
- 1 tbsp. olive oil
- 1/2 tsp. paprika
- 1/2 tsp. onion powder
- 1/2 tsp. garlic powder
- 1 medium onion
- 1/4 tsp. pepper
- 3/4 tsp. sea salt

Directions:

1. Slice onion and radishes using a mandolin slicer.
2. Add sliced onion and radishes in a large mixing bowl and toss with olive oil.
3. Transfer onion and radish slices in Air Fryer basket and cook at 360°F for 8 minutes Shake basket twice.

4. Return onion and radish slices in a mixing bowl and toss with seasonings.

5. Again, cook onion and radish slices in Air Fryer basket for 5 minutes at 400°F. Shake the basket halfway through.

6. Serve and enjoy.

Nutrition:

Calories 62, Fat 3.7g, Carbs 7.1g, Protein 1.2g

Vegetable Egg Cups

Preparation Time: 10 minutes

Cooking Time: 20 minutes

Servings: 4

Ingredients:

- 4 eggs
- 1 tbsp. cilantro, chopped
- 4 tbsp. half and half
- 1 cup cheddar cheese, shredded
- 1 cup vegetables, diced
- Pepper
- Salt

Directions:

1. Sprinkle four ramekins with cooking spray and set aside.
2. In a mixing bowl, whisk eggs with cilantro, half and half, vegetables, 1/2 cup cheese, pepper, and salt.
3. Pour egg mixture into the four ramekins.

4. Place ramekins in Air Fryer basket and cook at 300°F for 12 minutes
5. Top with remaining 1/2 cup cheese and cook for 2 minutes more at 400°F.
6. Serve and enjoy.

Nutrition:

Calories 194, Fat 11.5g, Carbs 6g, Protein 13g

Spinach Frittata

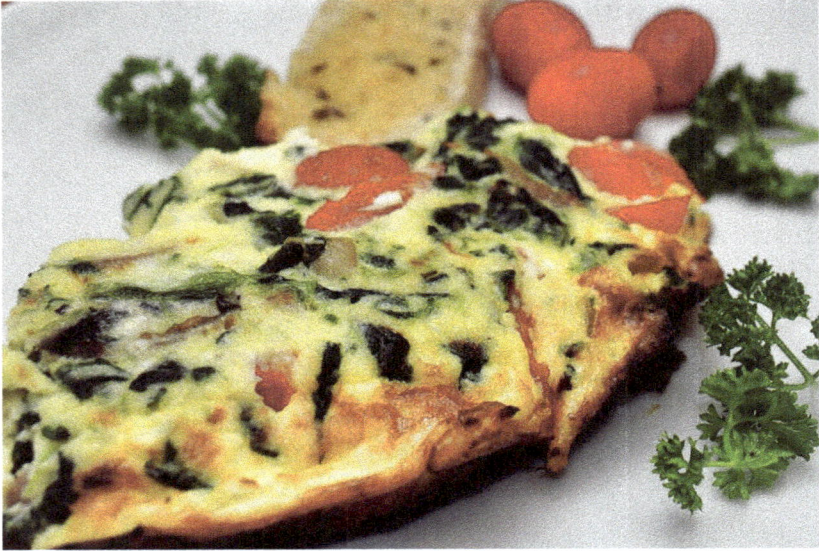

Preparation Time: 5 minutes

Cooking Time: 8 minutes

Servings: 1

Ingredients:

- 3 eggs
- 1 cup spinach, chopped
- 1 small onion, minced
- 2 tbsp. mozzarella cheese, grated

- Pepper
- Salt

Directions:

1. Preheat the Air Fryer to 350°F. Spray Air Fryer pan with cooking spray.
2. In a bowl, whisk eggs with remaining ingredients until well combined.
3. Pour egg mixture into the prepared pan and place pan in the Air Fryer basket.
4. Cook frittata for 8 minutes or until set. Serve and enjoy.

Nutrition:

Calories 384, Fat 23.3g, Carbs 10.7g, Protein 34.3g

Omelet Frittata

Preparation Time: 10 minutes

Cooking Time: 6 minutes

Servings: 2

Ingredients:

- 3 eggs, lightly beaten
- 2 tbsp. cheddar cheese, shredded
- 2 tbsp. heavy cream
- 2 mushrooms, sliced
- 1/4 small onion, chopped
- 1/4 bell pepper, diced
- Pepper
- Salt

Directions:

1. In a bowl, whisk eggs with cream, vegetables, pepper, and salt.
2. Preheat the Air Fryer to 400°F.
3. Pour egg mixture into the Air Fryer pan. Place pan in Air Fryer basket and cook for 5 minutes

4. Add shredded cheese on top of the frittata and cook for 1 minute more.

5. Serve and enjoy.

Nutrition:

Calories 160, Fat 10, Carbs 4g, Protein 12g

Cheese Soufflés

Preparation Time: 10 minutes

Cooking Time: 6 minutes

Servings: 8

Ingredients:

- 6 large eggs, separated
- 3/4 cup heavy cream
- 1/4 tsp. cayenne pepper
- 1/2 tsp. xanthan gum
- 1/2 tsp. pepper
- 1/4 tsp. cream of tartar
- 2 tbsp. chives, chopped
- 2 cups cheddar cheese, shredded
- 1 tsp. salt

Directions:

1. Preheat the Air Fryer to 325°F.
2. Spray eight ramekins with cooking spray. Set aside.
3. In a bowl, whisk together almond flour, cayenne pepper, pepper, salt, and xanthan gum.

4. Slowly add heavy cream and mix to combine.
5. Whisk in egg yolks, chives, and cheese until well combined.
6. In a large bowl, add egg whites and cream of tartar and beat until stiff peaks form.
7. Fold egg white mixture into the almond flour mixture until combined.
8. Pour mixture into the prepared ramekins. Divide ramekins in batches.
9. Place the first batch of ramekins into the Air Fryer basket.
10. Cook soufflé for 20 minutes
11. Serve and enjoy.

Nutrition:

Calories 210, Fat 16g, Carbs 1g, Protein 12g

Cheese and Red Pepper Egg Cups

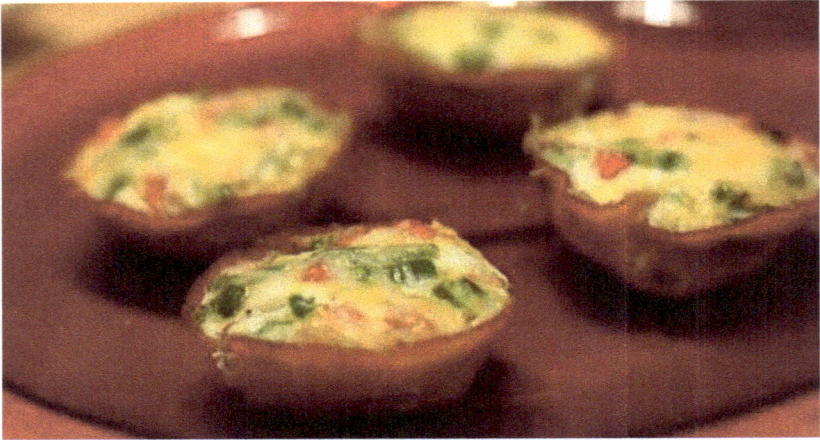

Preparation Time: 10 minutes

Cooking Time: 15 minutes

Servings: 4

Ingredients:

- 4 Large free-range eggs
- 1 cup Shredded cheese
- 1 cup Diced red pepper
- 4 tbsps half and half
- Salt and Pepper.

Directions:

1. Preheat your Air Fryer to 300°F and grease four ramekins.
2. Grab a medium bowl and add the eggs. Whisk well.
3. Add the red pepper, half the cheese, half and half, salt and pepper. Stir well to combine.
4. Pour the mixture between the ramekins and pop into the Air Fryer.
5. Cook for 15 minutes then serve and enjoy.

Nutrition:

Calories 195, Fat 12g, Carbs 7g, Protein 13g

Coconut Porridge with Flax Seed

Preparation Time: 5 minutes

Cooking Time: 30 minutes

Servings: 3

Ingredients:

- 1 ½ cup Unsweetened almond milk
- 2 tbsp. Coconut flour
- 2 tbsp. Vegan vanilla protein powder
- ¼ tsp. Powdered erythritol
- 3 tbsp. Golden flaxseed meal

Directions:

1. Preheat your Air Fryer at a temperature of about 375°F
2. Combine coconut flour with the golden flaxseed meal and the protein powder in a bowl
3. Spray your Air Fryer with cooking spray, then pour the mixture in the Air Fryer pan
4. Pour the milk and top with chopped blueberries and chopped raspberries

5. Move the pan in the Air Fryer and close
6. Set the temperature at about 375°F and the timer to about 30 minutes
7. When the timer beeps, turn off your Air Fryer and remove the baking pan
8. Serve and enjoy your delicious porridge!

Nutrition:

Calories 249, Fats 13.7g, Carbs 6g, Protein 17g

Easy Chocolate Doughnut

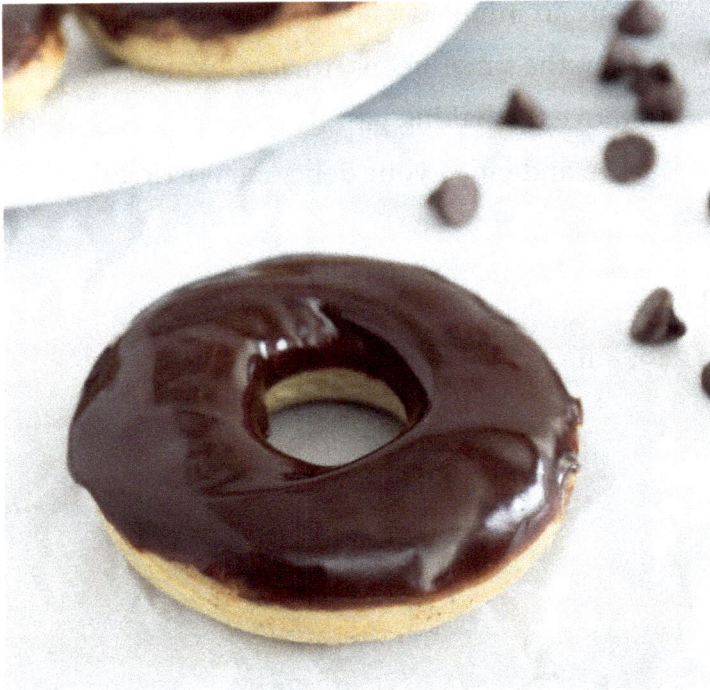

Preparation Time: 10 minutes

Cooking Time: 12 minutes

Servings: 6

Ingredients:

- 3 tbsps Melted unsalted butter
- ¼ cup Powdered sugar

- 8 Refrigerated biscuits
- 48 Semisweet chocolate chips

Directions:

1. Cut the biscuits into thirds then flatten them and place 2 chocolate chips at the center.
2. Wrap the chocolate with dough to seal the edges.
3. Rub each dough hole with some butter.
4. Set the dough into the Air Fryer to cook for 12 minutes at 340°F.
5. Set aside to add powdered sugar.
6. Serve and enjoy.

Nutrition:

Calories 393, Fat 17g, Carbs 55g, Protein 5g

Cheesy Spinach Omelet

Preparation Time: 5 minutes

Cooking Time: 10 minutes

Servings: 2

Ingredients

- 3 Eggs
- 2 tbsps Chopped fresh spinach
- ½ cup Shredded cheese
- Pepper
- Salt

Directions

1. Mix the eggs with pepper and salt then whisk and put in an oven-safe tray.
2. Add spinach and cheese but do not stir.
3. Allow to cook in the Air Fryer for 8 minutes at 390°F.
4. Cook for 2 more minutes to brown the omelet.
5. Serve on plates to enjoy.

Nutrition:

Calories 209, Fat 15.9g, Carbs 1g, Protein 15.4g

Roasted Garlic and Thyme Dipping Sauce

Preparation Time: 5 minutes

Cooking Time: 30 minutes

Servings: 1

Ingredients:

- ½ tsp. Minced fresh thyme leaves
- 1/8 tsp. Salt
- ½ cup Light mayonnaise
- 2 tbsps Crushed roasted garlic
- 1/8 tsp. Pepper

Directions:

1. Wrap garlic in foil. Put it in the cooking basket of the Air Fryer and roast for 30 minutes at 390°F.
2. Combine all the ingredients to serve.

Nutrition:

Calories 485, Fat 39.4g, Carbs 34.1g, Protein 2.2g

Cheesy Sausage and Egg Rolls

Preparation Time: 15 minutes

Cooking Time: 15 minutes

Servings: 8

Ingredients:

- 8 pieces Cooked breakfast sausage links
- 3 Eggs
- Salt and Pepper
- 4 Cheddar cheese slices
- 8 oz. Refrigerated crescent rolls

Directions:

1. Set the Air Fryer at 325°F to preheat.
2. Beat the eggs; reserve one tbsp. as egg wash and scramble the rest.
3. Halve the cheese slices. Separate the dough into 8 triangles.
4. Fill each triangle with a half-slice of cheese, a tbsp. of scrambled eggs, and a sausage link.

5. Loosely roll up all filled triangles before placing in the Air Fryer basket. Brush with the egg wash that was set aside and sprinkle all over with pepper and salt.
6. Cook for 15 minutes. Serve right away.

Nutrition:

Calories 270, Fat 20.0g, Protein 10.0g, Carbs 13.0g

Baked Berry Oatmeal

Preparation Time: 5 minutes

Cooking Time: 25 minutes

Servings: 2-4

Ingredients:

- 1 medium-size egg
- 1 cup of whole milk
- 1 cup of rolled oats
- 2½ tbsp. of brown sugar
- ½ tsp. of baking powder
- ½ tsp. of ground cinnamon
- Oil
- 2 cups of divided, mixed berries
- 2 tbsp. of slivered almonds
- Sprinkling of nutmeg

Directions:

1. In a bowl, combine the egg with the milk, mixing well to combine.

2. In a second bowl, combine the oats with the brown sugar, baking powder, and cinnamon. Mix thoroughly.
3. Spritz your Air Fryer safe pan with oil spray.
4. Add ¼ cup of the mixed berries to the Air Fryer.
5. Pour the oatmeal mixture over the fruit, followed by the egg and milk mixture.
6. Allow to rest for approximately 10 minutes before adding the remaining fruit on top.
7. Scatter the slivered almonds over the berries and season with a sprinkling of nutmeg.
8. Place the pan in your Air Fryer and bake at 320°F, for 10 minutes. Check the progress and either continue to bake or remove from the appliance.
9. Set aside to rest for 4-5 minutes and serve.

Nutrition:

Calories 151, Fat 7.1g, Carbs 17.9g, Protein 3.6g

Broccoli and Cheddar Cheese Quiche

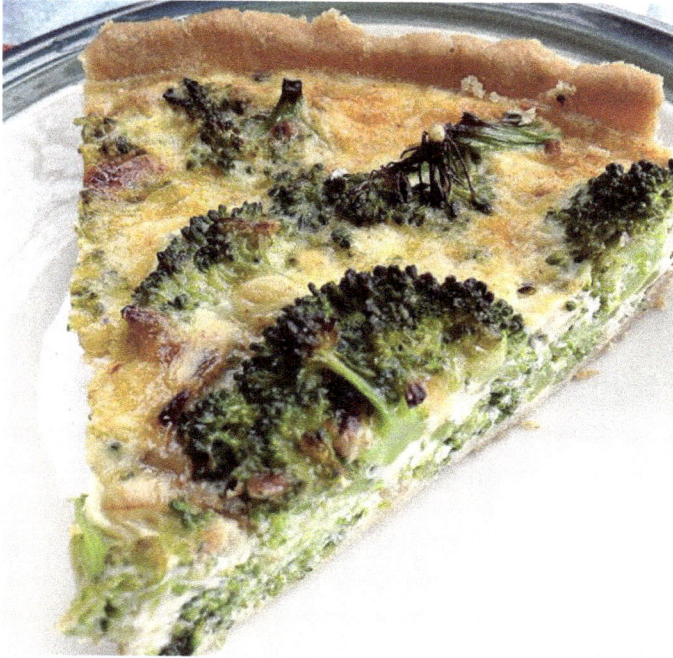

Preparation Time: 5 minutes

Cooking Time: 10 minutes

Servings: 1

Ingredients:

- 1 medium-size egg
- 3-4 tbsp. of heavy cream

- 4-5 very small-size broccoli florets
- 1 tbsp. of finely grated Cheddar cheese

Directions:

1. In a bowl, whisk the egg along with the heavy cream.
2. Lightly grease a 5" circular, ceramic quiche-style dish.
3. Arrange the broccoli florets evenly on the bottom of the dish.
4. Pour in the egg-cream mixture.
5. Scatter the grated Cheddar cheese over the top and air fry at 325°F for 10 minutes.
6. Serve and enjoy.

Nutrition:

Calories 162, Fat 5.23g, Carbs 14.3g, Protein 9.4g

Egg and Cheese Puff Pastry Tarts

Preparation Time: 10 minutes

Cooking Time: 20 minutes

Servings: 4

Ingredients:

- All-purpose flour
- 1 (9") square sheet of frozen, thawed puff pastry
- ¾ cup of shredded Cheddar cheese
- 4 large-size eggs
- 1 tbsp. of minced fresh chives

Directions:

1. Preheat the Air Fryer to 390°F.
2. On a lightly floured clean work surface, unfold the sheet of pastry and cut it into 4 even squares.
3. Put 2 of the pastry squares in the Air Fryer basket, spacing them apart from one another.
4. Air fry until the pastry is a light golden brown, for approximately 10 minutes.

5. Open the basket, and with a metal spoon, press down the middles of each pastry square to create an indentation. Scatter 3 tbsp. of shredded cheese into each indent. Crack an egg carefully into the middle of each pastry.
6. Air fry for 8-10 minutes, until the eggs are cooked to your preferred level of doneness.
7. Transfer the tarts to a wire baking rack set over wax paper and allow it to cool for 4-5 minutes.
8. Repeat Steps 2-4 with the remaining ingredients.
9. Garnish with half of the chives and serve warm.

Nutrition:

Calories 231, Fat 6.5g, Carbs 10.3g, Protein 6.4g

French Toast

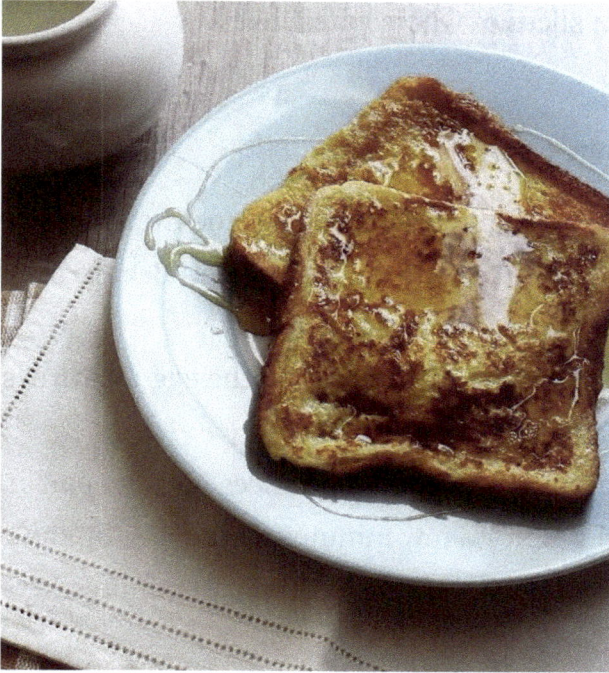

Preparation Time: 5 minutes

Cooking Time: 3 Minutes

Servings: 4

Ingredients:

- 2 medium-size eggs
- ⅔ cup of whole milk

- 1 tbsp. of cinnamon
- 1 tsp. of vanilla extract
- 4 slices of whole wheat bread

Directions:

1. In a small-size bowl, combine the eggs with the milk, cinnamon, and vanilla extract. Beat to break up the eggs and incorporate them.
2. Dip each side of bread in the egg mixture, shaking off any excess.
3. Add the dipped bread slices into the pan and Air Fryer for a few minutes at 320°F. Flip the bread over and air fry for an additional 3 minutes.
4. Serve.

Nutrition:

Calories 231, Fat 6.3g, Carbs 13.6g, Protein 4.6g

Grilled Gruyere Cheese Sandwich

Preparation Time: 5 minutes

Cooking Time: 10 minutes

Servings: 1

Ingredients:

- 2 oz. of thinly sliced Gruyere cheese
- 2 slices of whole-grain bread
- 1 tbsp. of butter

Directions:

1. Lay the Gruyere cheese between the 2 slices of bread.
2. Butter up the outside of the bread slices.
3. Place the cheese sandwich in the Air Fryer basket. You may need to use toothpicks to secure.
4. Air fry the sandwich for approximately 3-5 minutes at 360°F until the cheese melts.
5. Flip the sandwich over and turn the heat up to 380°F until crisp.
6. Continue to Air Fryer for approximately 5 minutes, until the sandwich is to your desired texture. You will

need to check continually that the sandwich doesn't burn.

7. Set to one side to cool slightly before enjoying.

Nutrition:

Calories 151, Fat 7.1g, Carbs 17.9g, Protein 3.6g

Pancakes

Preparation Time: 5 minutes

Cooking Time: 10 minutes

Servings: 2

Ingredients:

- 2 tbsps. coconut oil
- 1 tsp. maple extract
- 2 tbsps. cashew milk
- 2 eggs
- 2/3 oz. /20g pork rinds

Directions:

1. Grind up the pork rinds until fine and mix with the rest of the ingredients, except the oil.
2. Add the oil to a skillet. Add a quarter-cup of the batter and fry until golden on each side. Continue adding the remaining batter.

Nutrition:

Calories 280, Carbs 31g, Fat 2g, Protein 5g

Breakfast Sandwich

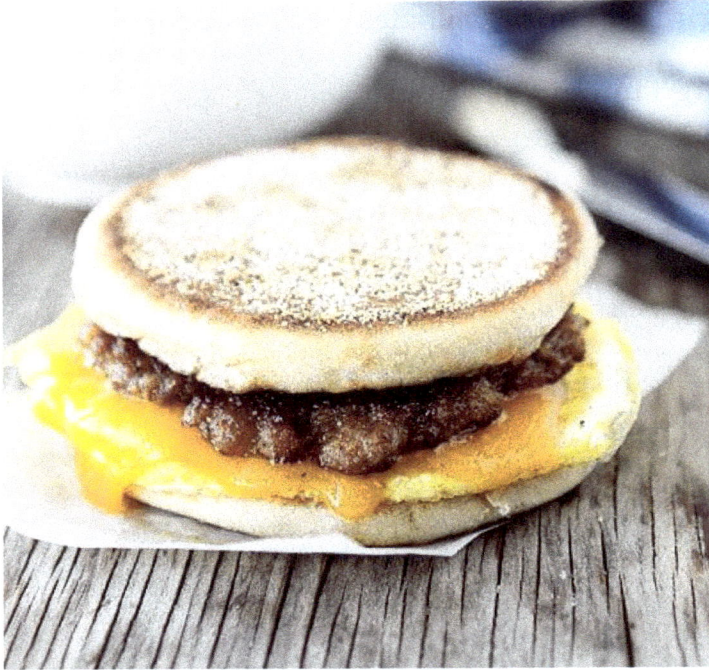

Preparation Time: 5 minutes

Cooking Time: 5 minutes

Servings: 2

Ingredients:

- 2 oz. /60g cheddar cheese
- 1/6 oz. /30g smoked ham

- 2 tbsps. butter
- 4 eggs

Directions:

1. Spray your Air Fryer pan with olive oil. Crack the eggs into the pan
2. Air fry for 3 minutes at 370°F, sprinkle pepper and salt on them.
3. Place an egg down as the sandwich base. Top with the ham and cheese and a drop or two of Tabasco.
4. Place the other egg on top and enjoy.

Nutrition:

Calories 180, Carbs 19g, Fat 7g, Protein 10g

Egg Muffins

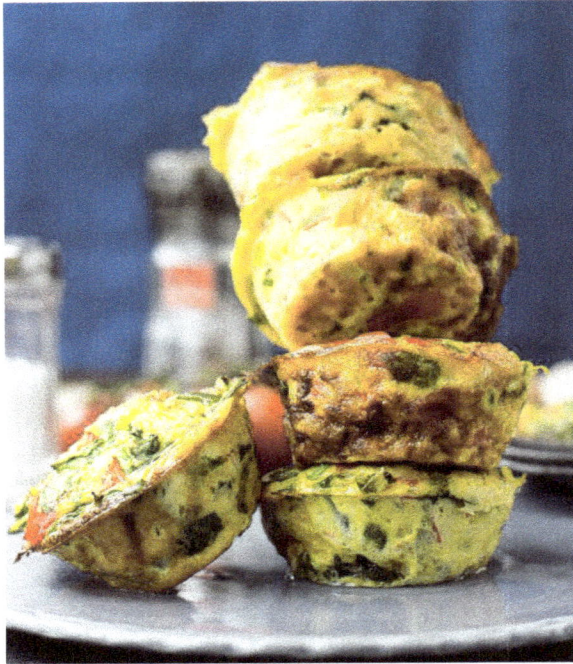

Preparation Time: 10 minutes

Cooking Time: 15-20 minutes

Servings: 4

Ingredients:

- 1 tbsp. green pesto
- 1/3 cup of shredded cheese

- 1/3 cup of cooked bacon
- 1 scallion, chopped
- 6 Eggs

Directions:

1. You should set your fryer to 350°F.
2. Place liners in a regular cupcake tin. This will help with easy removal and storage.
3. Beat the eggs with pepper, salt, and the pesto. Mix in the cheese.
4. Pour the eggs into the cupcake tin and top with the bacon and scallion.
5. Cook for 15-20 minutes, or until the egg is set.

Nutrition:

Calories 16, Carbs 11g, Fat 6g, Protein 8g

Bacon & Eggs

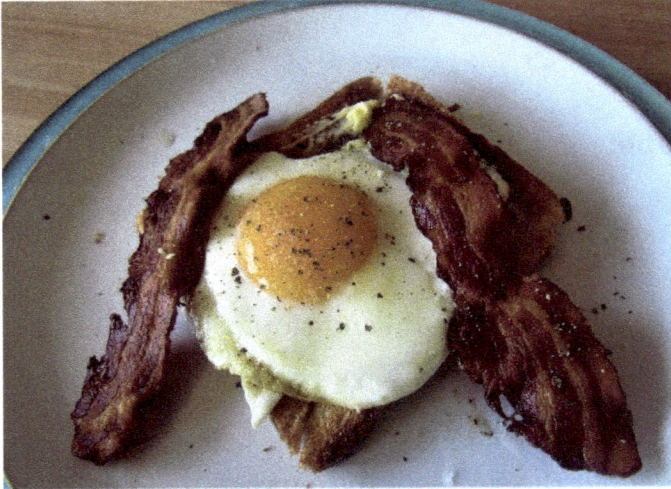

Preparation Time: 5 minutes

Cooking Time: 5 minutes

Servings: 4

Ingredients:

- Parsley
- Cherry tomatoes
- 1/3 oz. /150g bacon
- 6 Eggs

Directions:

1. Set your air Fryer at 370°F. Fry up the bacon for 5 minutes and put it to the side with the grease.
2. Spray your Air Fryer pan with olive oil. Crack the eggs into the pan
3. Air fry for 3 minutes at 370°F, sprinkle pepper and salt on them
4. Scramble the eggs in the bacon grease, with some pepper and salt. If you want, scramble in some cherry tomatoes. Sprinkle with some parsley and enjoy.

Nutrition:

Calories 150, Carbs 10g, Fat 6g, Protein 7g

Eggs on the Go

Preparation Time: 5 minutes

Cooking Time: 15 minutes

Servings: 1

Ingredients:

- 110g bacon, cooked
- Pepper
- Salt
- 6 Eggs

Directions:

1. You should set your fryer to 370°F.
2. Place liners in a regular cupcake tin. This will help with easy removal and storage.
3. Crack an egg into each of the cups and sprinkle some bacon onto each of them. Season with some pepper and salt.
4. Bake for 15 minutes, or once the eggs are set.

Nutrition:

Calories 140, Carbs 10g, Fat 5g, Protein 7g

Protein Banana Bread

Preparation Time: 10 minutes

Cooking Time: 1 hour 10 minutes

Servings: 16

Ingredients:

- 3 eggs
- 1/3 cup coconut flour
- 1/2 cup swerve
- 2 cups almond flour
- 1/2 cup ground chia seed
- 1/2 tsp. vanilla extract
- 4 tbsp. butter, melted
- 3/4 cup almond milk
- 1 tbsp. baking powder
- 1/3 cup protein powder
- 1/2 cup water
- 1/2 tsp. salt

Directions:

1. Grease loaf pan with butter and set aside.

2. Set temperature 325°F, timer for 1 hour 10 minutes. Press start to preheat the Air Fryer.

3. In a small bowl, whisk together chia seed and 1/2 cup water. Set aside.

4. In a large bowl, mix together almond flour, baking powder, protein powder, coconut flour, sweetener, and salt.

5. Stir in eggs, milk, chia seed mixture, vanilla extract, and butter until well combined.

6. Pour batter into the prepared loaf pan and bake for 1 hour 10 minutes.

7. Sliced and serve.

Nutrition:

Calories 162, Carbs 13.4g, Fat 11.2g, Protein 5.2g

Easy Kale Muffins

Preparation Time: 10 minutes

Cooking Time: 30 minutes

Servings: 8

Ingredients:

- 6 eggs
- 1/2 cup milk
- 1/4 cup chives, chopped
- 1 cup kale, chopped
- Salt and Pepper

Directions:

1. Spray 8 cups muffin pan with cooking spray and set aside.
2. Set temperature 350°F, timer for 30 minutes. Press start to preheat the Air Fryer.
3. Add all ingredients into the mixing bowl and whisk well.
4. Pour mixture into the prepared muffin pan and bake for 30 minutes.

5. Serve and enjoy.

Nutrition:

Calories 89, Carbs 2g, Fat 3.6g, Protein 5g

Mozzarella Spinach Quiche

Preparation Time: 10 minutes

Cooking Time: 45 minutes

Servings: 6

Ingredients:

- 4 eggs
- 10 oz frozen spinach, thawed
- 1/2 cup mozzarella cheese, shredded
- 1/4 cup parmesan cheese, grated
- 8 oz mushrooms, sliced
- 2 oz feta cheese, crumbled
- 1 cup almond milk
- 1 garlic clove, minced
- Salt and Pepper

Directions:

1. Spray a pie dish with cooking spray and set aside.
2. Set temperature 350°F, timer for 45 minutes. Press start to preheat the Air Fryer.

3. Spray medium pan with cooking spray and heat over medium heat.
4. Add garlic, mushrooms, pepper, and salt in a pan and sauté for 5 minutes.
5. Add spinach in pie dish then add sautéed mushroom on top of spinach.
6. Sprinkle feta cheese over spinach and mushroom.
7. In a bowl, whisk eggs, parmesan cheese, and almond milk.
8. Pour egg mixture over spinach and mushroom then sprinkle shredded mozzarella cheese and bake for 45 minutes.
9. Sliced and serve.

Nutrition:

Calories 197, Carbs 6.2g, Fat 16g, Protein 10.4g

Fancy Breakfast Quinoa

Preparation Time: 10 minutes

Cooking Time: 3 Minutes

Serving: 4

Ingredients:

- 1/2 cup walnuts, soaked and chopped
- 4 oz. sesame seeds, soaked
- 2 oz. hemp seeds, soaked overnight
- 1 tsp. date sugar
- 1/2 tsp. ground cinnamon
- 5 oz. quinoa puff
- 1 tsp. hemp seed oil
- 1 cup of coconut milk

Directions:

1. Take a bowl and mix in all the seeds and spices. Add hemp seed oil
2. Stir well until the mixture is thick. Flatten mixture on your cooking basket
3. Preheat your Air Fryer to 330°F

4. Transfer to your Air Fryer and cook for 2-3 minutes until light brown
5. Transfer mix to a serving bowl. Add quinoa puff, stir well and add coconut milk stir again
6. Serve and enjoy

Nutrition:

Calories 510, Carbs 50 g, Fat 8g, Protein 21g

Fresh Sautéed Apple

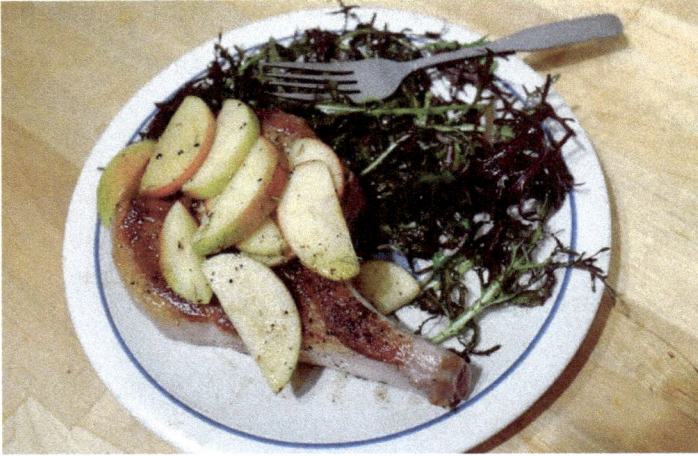

Preparation Time: 10 minutes

Cooking Time: 10 minutes

Serving: 4

Ingredients:

- 2 tbsp. olive oil
- 3 apples, peeled, cored and sliced
- 1 tbsp. garlic clove, grated
- 1 tbsp. date sugar
- Pinch of salt

Directions:

1. Preheat your Air Fryer 300°F. Add coconut oil to the cooking basket, add remaining ingredients and stir well.
2. Transfer to Air Fryer, cook for 5-10 minutes, making sure to shake the basket occasionally until golden. Serve and enjoy!

Nutrition:

Calories 32, Carbs 32g, Fat 9g, Protein 3g

www.ingramcontent.com/pod-product-compliance
Lightning Source LLC
Chambersburg PA
CBHW070736030426
42336CB00013B/1984